I0756586

SNORING THE ENIGMA- THE REAL REASONS AND THE ULTIMATE CURE TO STOP SNORING

Contents

Introduction

LAUGH AND THE WORLD LAUGHS WITH YOU, SNORE AND YOU SLEEP ALONE.

-Anthony Burgess

Here you go! Once again, you woke up to an empty bed. You climb out of bed and feel miserable. Tramping towards the kitchen, you pass the living room and see your significant half lying on the couch sleeping. Again!

You can't deny it; you are well aware that you're doing it. The love of your life has all the evidence of the nocturnal noises you make. But you just can't seem to stop it.

For you, it might be embarrassing when your partner rags on you about your thumping snoring and a whole lot worse when your kids make fun of the roaring jet engine sounds you make all through the night. But now you say to yourself, that's it! That recording of you snorting like a horse was all you needed to take it seriously and do something to make the life of your loved ones a tad bit easier.

Now that you have accepted that there is an issue that is fostering within you, you make a promise to your loved ones that you will make your place in the list of the non-snorers of the house. You see, everyone elated and dancing with joy to finally have peaceful nights and feel yourself like a hero for making their day. Does the story sound too good to be true? What do you think?

Snoring has been identified as a common disorder that can affect anyone, either men or women. Look around in your circle and spot the snorers you have in your group. Just about everyone in your group snores[1]. If we dig deeper, we find that snoring is a kind of medical condition or a health issue that occurs when the air is blocked.

Itis not only a cause of annoyance for others, but it also impairs the person's own sleep as well. This trumpeting, rumbling, thumping, and echoing sound can keep the person himself and others around him, awake all through the night. It can easily disrupt your sleep leading to fatigue, poor health, tiredness, and irritability. While some say snoring is just another hint that you are getting old, others are of the opinion that it can hit anyone as it's believed to be a medical condition.

The story of snoring continues! But quitting snoring is not as simple as snapping your fingers. It is a time consuming and tedious process that requires totally patience and dedication. There are several strategies, cures, and remedies that claim to reduce snoring;

some even claim to put an end to it for as long as you shall live. But all these remedies and strategies can only be tried out after you discover the real cause of your snoring.

It is high time that we treat this nuisance since it has become a pain in the neck of many. It is also becoming a real cause of splitting up or even leading to divorces between couples[2]. Besides, it is not just a means of embarrassment; it might be indicating a serious medical issue that needs attention or requires a change in your lifestyle. Ignoring symptoms can lead to serious health risks and damage the body in the long term.

This is precisely where this book can help you with. You will bust the myths about snoring, uncover its secrets, and will find ways to decode those secrets. This book will enlighten you with the remedies of snoring while helping you with pointing out its real causes. From ancient ones to the modern tried and tested all the way to prove ones scientifically, this book contains tongue workouts, recommendations for buying the right gadgets, and an overview of what to do if nothing of this works. Whether young or old, male or female, thin or fat, in the end you know the difference between harmless snoring and serious medical problems.

I hope you will learn a lot on your journey and wish you good luck to beat your snoring once and for all!

Understanding the enigma of snoring

-Judy Blume

We all have heard many myths about snoring. While some are identified as 'old wives' tales', others are found to be true and especially dangerous to our health. For example, snoring is often believed to be a comical thing, as portrayed in movies and television. Even in real life, we make fun of the ones who snore around us. We tell you, it doesn't feel good at all. Unless you have ever snored or experienced living with a bed partner who snores, you couldn't know how it feels. It's annoying, frustrating, and somewhat embarrassing, isn't it?

According to National Sleep Foundation statistics, around 1 in 3 men and 1 in 4 women snore while they sleep every night[3]. The statistical result shows that it is a common companion of many people. Almost 90 million Americans are affected by snoring. The clinical name of snoring is "stertor"; the literal meaning of this word is *'loud, raspy, laboured breathing, caused by obstructed respiratory passages'*. This word is derived from the Latin word *stert(ere)* and was first used in 1804. Today it occurs to all sorts of people, regardless of their age or sex.

In medical terms, it is the vibration of the respiratory structure caused by the obstruction in the passage of air through the nose and throat[4]. When the air is blocked physically through the mouth and nose, that's when snoring occurs. The area at the back of the throat narrows, its muscles relax or sometimes temporarily close off when we sleep. The air passing through the small opening rapidly can cause the tissues surrounding the opening to vibrate, which can cause the sounds of snoring[5].

This sound is like any other vibration sound, for example: When we speak, our vocal cords vibrate and hence produce a sound. Take a look at another example; we all experience stomach growling occasionally. When air and food pass through our intestines, our stomach growls similarly; when one draws a breath, it occurs while it may also happen when they breathe out[6]. Each one of us occasionally snores, while some people are soft snorers, many others snore chronically.

Why people snore?

Dr. Brett Comer, a head and neck surgeon, as well as an associate professor of Otolaryngology at the University of Kentucky, says: 'We tend to lose muscle tone when we're asleep - this way, the tongue flops back and the tissues and muscles in the throat and nose relax. There are a bunch of other factors, too, that play a noteworthy role in a person's propensity to snore. Overweight, indulgence in alcohol, and sleeping on your back are a few to name[7]. I will explain the causes later.

Some reasons to snore may sound like a myth, often a few others are discovered as a real cause of this headache. The most common reason that you will probably come across every time you hear or read the word of snoring is sleep apnea. To find out why 'snoring' and sleep apnea are used interchangeably, let's dive straight into what it is[8].

Sleep Apnea - why every discussion on snoring leads to sleep apnea?

From a medical perspective, snoring could be a sign of a chronic condition. Distinguishing between snoring and sleep apnea is the key to treat the condition. While snoring is just a vibration, creating a sound, loud and frequent snores hint towards sleep apnea or Obstructive Sleep Apnea[9]. There are two types of apnea:

Obstructive Sleep Apnea (OSA)

The blockage or pauses in breathing caused due to the collapse or narrowing of the upper airway is known as Obstructive Sleep Apnea. It usually causes the person to wake up to breathe again. This doesn't happen in regular snoring. OSA obstruction is hard on the chest and diaphragm muscles, causing them to work up to open the blocked airway. This is the most common type of apnea.

Central sleep apnea (CSA)

This type of sleep apnea doesn't block the airway, but due to the fragility in the respiratory system, the brain fails to send signals to the muscles to breathe. Central Sleep Apnea is associated with severe illness in which the lower brain is affected[10]. This type is not very commonly found in people.

Who snores?

A MARRIAGE IS ALWAYS MADE UP OF TWO PEOPLE WHO ARE PREPARED TO SWEAR
THAT ONLY THE OTHER ONE SNORES.

-Terry Pratchett

Winston Churchill was an infamous snorer. And so was Queen Victoria, allegedly[20].When it comes to snoring, we usually picture a large-sized guy with his massive body stretched out on the bed, creating thumping and thwacking sounds out of his nostrils and mouth. But that's not always true! A tall, slender, and graceful lady can snore just as loudly. And some people are so boisterous that you can literally hear their energy in the form of snores.

According to National Sleep Foundation statistics, around 1 in 3 men and 1 in 4 women snore every night[21]. Regardless of gender, snoring can start at any age. However, it's not normal to snore at any age[22].

As we age, we are literally stormed by health issues. Your greying hair is a sign that you are now more prone to a variety of illnesses and medical conditions. The problem of snoring responds no difference to this natural process of ageing. In all honesty, it elevates with age. Occasional snorers become regular and frequent snorers, regardless of their gender[23].

To receive an even clearer picture of what happens to our snoring habits as we age, we first need to understand the changes that occur in our body and sleeping patterns as we grow older.

Ageing and snoring – the sweet old relationship

With every tick of the clock, we lose a second of our life. As humans grow old, their physiology changes. As physiology of the human body changes, it starts to function differently, or should we say a little weird. We lose our appetite, our sleeping lessens, and our energy level declines[24].

Remember your granny singing lullabies and reading out bedtime stories to you? That's because they find it harder to sleep immediately in dotage[25]and sometimes stay up all night. Hence, they are more likely to snore.

As quoted in snore lab, no less than 10% of 17-29 years old say they frequently snore, while more than 40% of over 50 years of age do[26]. Snoring is so prevalent that people have found ways to profit from it. Now you know why you see so many customized pillows in the market with snoring written in bold.

It's inevitable to stop ageing, but it shouldn't be the same with snoring. So, what exactly is the relationship between age and snoring? Well, this time around, we don't have good news for you. Ageing actually affects the habit of snoring. It poses both direct and indirect causes.

Frail airway

Reality check for all! Have you ever closely observed the older people? It's not just that their patience has grown thin, but their skin as well from being thick, elastic, and supple. A major reason for such physical and internal changes is that their organs have started to shrink. This is a direct cause.

When the skin loses its tension and rigidity, the muscles of our body start to fatigue and become less toned. The tissues of our air passage begin to vibrate and lose its firmness. Therefore, this serves as a direct reason for snoring when a person becomes older.

There are some other indirect factors, too, that come with ageing, and they also play a vital part in turning you into a loud snorer. These include:

Gaining weight

Heads up, you chubby fellas! Check your weight. If the needle of the weighing machine budges at a stroke, know that it's an indication. Carrying excess weight on your body not only adversely affects your health, also it can lead towards harsh snoring[27]. Here you might find yourself wondering, what is excess weight? Excess weight is having more body fat than is optimally healthy. Excess weight can be found by calculating the BMI.

Body Mass Index (BMI)

is a measure of body size in relation to the height of the body. It calculates points out of height and weight and is only a rough standard[28]. The screening tool can indicate whether a person is underweight, overweight if they have a healthy weight, or obese. You fall within the underweight range if your BMI is less than 18.5; if it's 18.5 to 24.9, you fall within the normal or Healthy Weight range. In case you are overweight, your BMI will be between 25.0 and 29.9. If your BMI is 30.0 or exceeds, you fall within the obese range[29].

Many studies have been conducted on the relationship between BMI and snoring. And most of the studies showed that people with high Body Mass Index (BMI) are at higher risk of snoring and other sleep disorders[30].

Much as slumping against the cushions may always tempt you; reduced physical activity can drag you to snore heavily[31]. Moreover, less exertion and slow metabolism rate make age and weight gain go hand in hand. We tend to store fat on different body parts due to less muscular movements, particularly weight gained on the neck and midriff worsens the risk of snoring.

Breaking a sweat can help you accomplish to eliminate those nocturnal sounds you make.

Use of medication

Check your medicinal pouch and see the number of pills you swallow in a day. If the number is more than 10, then you may need to consult your doctor and tell them to prescribe you only the most important ones.[32]

Medications and other drugs used to treat medical issues such as high blood pressure; heart conditions can lead to a congested nose, which makes snoring chronic[33]. If you are too tired and want your muscles to loosen up a little, don't go for tranquilizers and muscle relaxants as they also increase the chances of snoring[34].

Declining immunity

It is not necessary that this only happens as you grow old. Our immune system responds to ageing the same way as any other system of our body; that is, it also gets weaker with time. We tend to have a more clogged nose and throat infections, which are often the result of us catches a cold. Having a clogged nose means loud and harsh snores, and this is why people snore more as they age.

At this point, some of you might be wondering that you are full of youth and have none of these issues still, how come your snore sounds like a jet engine just ready to take off? Stop stirring your thoughts; it's too hasty for conclusions. There can be some other reasons too apart from ageing. Time to flip the picture and look at the other aspect of your life too. Your lifestyle!

Ageing is inevitable, but to everyone's surprise, the problem does not only affect older people. A mass of youngsters also struggles with this problem.

Yes, fewer young people also snore in comparison to the older population, but this term, "fewer" still make up hundreds and thousands of adults[35]. There are a number of other culprits we can blame for creating this nuisance. We are progressively seeing that snoring and sleep apnea is a problem not only for older people but for youngsters and children as well.

Looking at the bigger picture, sometimes, it is the daily choices that we make which contribute to our health and issues related to it. Your lifestyle choices and daily routine can attribute considerably to snoring. Four of such major choices you make are:

Dehydration

Not drinking enough water is one of such bad choices. Recall your primary grade science class when you would see a picture of the human body with a teacher telling you what percentage of your body is made up of water. Up to 60% of the human body is water. If you don't drink enough water throughout the day, your inner organs can dry out, making your nasal and mouth dry too causing you to experience loud nightly disruptions[36].

Sleep deprivation

Like late-night parties and chatting with your buddies? We know the answer. It is the second-worst choice that we make. Yes, the myth that we snore more when we are in a deep sleep is true in some cases. The more tired you are, the more likely you are to disturb people around you with snores. Try to take seven to eight hours of sleep every day[37]. Else you will end up snoring like a grizzly bear.

Obesity

Occasionally we all love to binge eat. And on weekends, adults like to party and make frequent visits to the refrigerator all night long. Though that ice-cream tub full of chocolate chips resting in the freezer is enticing you to devour it. Know that being a snorer and being obese are linked together. Obesity and snoring go hand in hand. Carrying those extra pounds on your body not only adversely affects one's health, but it can even add up to the odds of snoring. Weight loss might be the most effective remedy to stop snoring.

Shedding off those extra pounds will not only make you look gorgeous but can help considerably with your snoring habit.

Alcohol, booze & tobacco

As they say: *"You look like what you put (eat) in your body."*
You wake up looking like a mess the next morning when you spent the other night partying and downing a few drinks, don't you?

Remember that a few drinks will make it worse. The use of alcohol and tobacco are major contributors. While alcohol acts as a tranquilizer for the muscles around the throat, smoke triggers irritation and inflammation in the airways. And a mix of both can cause snoring to be harsher, louder, and more frequent[38].

If a snoring battle is raging in your bedroom, know that you're not alone. The good news is that now you know a tad bit more about snoring, so you can always make a few changes to your lifestyle that may lower your risk of snoring. If you have tried all of the above tips and snoring persists, there's no need to freak out because there are still a few chapters left to read. Hang on!

We have a lot of reasons of what causes snoring. It would be easy, if you knew that you should just stop smoking. But what if it's more complex? What if the reason is your gender? Let's have a look in the next chapter for reasons, that you cannot change that easily.

Medical conditions and causes triggering snoring

After a tiring day at work, when you come back home, all you want to have is a peaceful night's sleep. However, often it seems like a fantasy when your snoring partner is around. Many of us have been robbed of a good night's sleep or been banished to another room because of snoring at some point in our life.

Often the snorer in the family has been the laughingstock. From being likened to a train engine to a faulty lawnmower, snorers find themselves on the receiving end. But what if we tell you that snoring goes way beyond just those seemingly comical loud noises? It might be alarming for some people to discover that snoring is not just another common disorder. It can be a serious indication of a crippling illness that needs to be treated as soon as possible.

Though snores feel like mere sounds, this annoyance has been able to attract the attention of the researchers. To decipher this enigma, many studies have been conducted on snoring, and most of them have revealed that the phenomenon of snoring is related to certain health issues apart from other common factors. While some of these causes aren't any cause for a concern, there are a few conditions, which require immediate attention and medical assistance.

Some of you may fear to read on the remaining book, but it is just to let you know how fit and healthy you are and where you stand with this problem. Take a dive into the less typical and unheard causes of snoring.

Gender

A Study in Switzerland from 2019 shows that men have more long-term problems with snoring than women. The Review paper shows, the Heartbeats are more irregular overnight, if you are a snorer and additionally a man. So, in conclusion, a male has more health risks as a snorer than a female[40].

Pregnancy

It's the news you have been waiting for months or probably years. You are on the moon after hearing it. But wait! Is your wife's snoring all through this time is making you go all crazy? Well, this time around, you have to endure it.

Snoring is fairly normal during pregnancy, even if you've never snored before. The most probable culprits of snoring in pregnant women are their surging pregnancy hormones as they become the reason for mucous membranes in the nose to swell, causing nasal congestions that surge up when you lie down. Also, the increase in abdominal girth and the uterus compressing on the diaphragm is to be blamed for your wife's snoring.

Heart disease or high cholesterol levels

Low-density lipoprotein (LDL), sometimes called 'bad' cholesterol, makes up most of your body's cholesterol. It is often associated with harmful effects on one's health and raises your risk of heart stroke. It is constituted of more fat than protein. An excess level of fat can amass and form lipid plaques in your arteries, leading to many heart diseases. According to the latest findings, having less than five hours of sleep can increase your LDL cholesterol levels and take you towards sleep apnea[41]. Individuals who sleep less pose a greater risk of having high cholesterol levels, and the odds of them snoring are high[42].

Allergies, congestion and your nasal structure

Now, let's try to understand the anatomy of our nose. Anything that causes an obstruction in breathing from the nose will have you snore. The wheezing sound that you sometimes hear when they are sleeping is also due to congestion of chest. Some individuals only snore when they have a sinus infection (nose congestion from a cold or flu), or during the allergy seasons. Deformities of nasal structure can also cause obstruction in breathing[43].

Abnormality in the carotid artery

According to Medical News Today, surgeons have found that there is an abnormality (thickening) in the carotid arteries of snorers as compared to non-snorers[44]. These medical terms may jiggle your brain cells a bit. However, it is important to know about them to get rid of your problem once and for all.

Basically, carotid arteries are the major vessels in the neck that carry oxygenated blood to the brain, face, and neck. The initial signs of carotid artery disease are Intima-media thickness. It is the measure of thickness of the two innermost layers of the wall of an artery.

Snorers have been found to have greater intima-media thickness. This malformation in snorers is now believed to be a real cause of snoring.

Genetic factors

If you are a habitual snorer and have tried all the hacks and tricks without much luck, this may indicate that your forefathers are to blame. Yes, snoring can have hereditary roots. Take a look at your family members and spot the snorers out there. If there are plenty of snorers in your family, especially your ancestors, then congratulations! You've been passed on the rather unwanted and quite unnecessary legacy of snoring.

These medical reasons aren't mentioned to scare you away! In fact, these are elaborated to give you knowledge about where you stand with your problem. It is always advised to check-in or have an appointment with your doctor if you have concerns about your health. A quick blood test is the most suitable option for those who are having such chronic issues of snoring. It can tell a lot about your well-being without burning a hole in your pocket.

To whip your system back into shape, there is nothing better than your doctor's advice and suggestions at this time. He can point you in the right direction. So, consult your family doctor and listen to them because medical conditions can only be cured through medical treatment!

So, there are little sins in our life that we can change and medical conditions, which needs medical treatment. In the next chapter I will explain some workouts that might help you with your issue.

Remedies and exercises to stop snoring

-Gene Tunney

As much as you want your snoring to stop, we are sure that your bed partner wants it even more than you. There are enough reasons to treat snoring. This sleep disturbing and irritating disorder is a giant hurdle in your good night's sleep[45]. Even if your snoring isn't personally keeping you up at night, it's an embarrassing condition that can make us nervous about sharing our bed with anyone. While we all need a good night's sleep, including the non-snoring partner, if you can't sleep due to snoring, it can lead to some serious health problems[46]. And you need to put an end to it.

For those who live in a hostel or dorm and have a habit of snoring, your bed partner or roommate can get frustrated and irritated and may even request to change their room. Imagine how mortifying it would be to let the whole management of your dorm know that you snore! And for those who live alone, well then, all such if you keep an eye on your health and notice any unusual symptoms such as dry mouth, waking up suddenly (not from a nightmare), feeling tired and having a headache.

Here's the good news! Gratefully, there are many remedies and exercises other than the chemist's shelf solutions, which people can try out first to reduce snoring noticeably. Scientists from Berlin tried to help snoring people with electro muscular training. It helped them to breath better at night, and even mild snorers got cured! The test persons trained for 20 minutes twice a day, over 8 weeks. So, you need to train constantly to gain any effects[47]. Try the following remedies and exercises, they are free, simple and a few of the exercises are even making fun.

Remedies

At first, we can try out some simple bedtime home remedies. It is important to keep in mind that though not all remedies are for everyone. For those who are single, which most of us are, and don't even have a bed partner, there are many apps through which they can keep track of their snoring and even check if they snore at all. These apps allow you to record, measure, and track your snoring, allowing you to discover ways to treat and reduce it. Some of the best apps include; *Sore lab, Snore report, Sleep talk, Snore recorder, and Snore Clock.* After keeping a track of your sleeping habits, you can try out these quick remedies and check later if this helped or not.

It is important to keep in mind that getting rid of snoring permanently requires persistence, changes in certain lifestyle habits, and willingness to try out different hacks[48].

Changing your normal daily posture to another one can be of help. Sleeping somewhere away from where you normally sleep may disrupt your snorting habit. If changing the position makes no sense to you, you can even try out to elevate your head a few inches. This will ease your breathing and flow of air through the airway. Also, there are specifically designed pillows such as Anti-snore pillow, Smart Nora, Nitetronic Goodnite level sleep restore pillow, InteVision foam wedge bed pillow available in the market to help prevent snoring by making sure your neck muscles are not crumpled[49.]Try side sleeping; this might just do the trick if your snoring is not as big of a problem. Sleeping on your side can avert the untoned neck muscles from blocking the air passage[50]. The problem is how to keep you on your side? Here's another oldie to try for you; attach a tennis ball to the back of your pajamas or back of your top. The discomfort of the ball will turn back to your side position.

Many people snore due to the dryness of the nose and mouth; a humidifier can help you with maintaining humidity in the air. Dry air causes irritation in the nose and throat, resulting in loud snorts and grunts during night time. Because we sleep the longest during the night, this trick might help stop snoring[51].

Stuffy nose and chest congestions trigger snoring, converting them into sounds like snorts even if it isn't sleeping apnea. It is better to clean your nose with saline water before jumping into bed. Try using peppermint oil also. It's found to be useful for sore throat relief and nose congestions[52]. Has your snoring stopped? This means you need to check that you don't sleep with a stuffy nose anymore.

The culture of being awake the whole night is not new to us. All of us like to party hard till late in the night and then drift to sleep as soon as it is over. Being awake the whole night and partying increases your chance of gorging on food. According to Snoring Source, consuming dairy products or large portions of the meal just before bedtime say like an hour before; can worsen snoring[53].

Working up a sweat can help us shed that extra weight around our belly. That's cool! But did you know that it can also help in putting a stop to your snoring? There are some exercises too, that can tackle snoring[54]. These highly focused stop snoring exercises are likely just the thing for you if you are looking for typical anti-snoring exercises. But here you are not doing squats or lunges! Instead, you are training and toning your mouth and throat muscles to stop making horrific noises[55].

Some specific exercises greatly contribute to toning and strengthening the muscles of the throat.

1. **Tongue curlers**

    Keep your mouth open and curl your tongue against the hard roof palate. Take your tongue as far back as it can go. Repeat it 20 times, and you'll see the difference in your snoring.

2. **Pronounce vowels**

    It is as simple as it sounds. Take your inner child out and imagine it's your grammar class. Repeat each vowel (a-e-i-o-u) aloud for two to three minutes a few times a day and hold for a few seconds while pronouncing each vowel. It's also a great way to teach your little one all the vowels.

3. **Shut your mouth**

    No, it's not like someone telling you to shut your mouth and mind your own business. It's an exercise to help you lessen the intensity of your snoring. Close your mouth for a few minutes, and purse your lips. Hold this position for 30 seconds.

4. **Move your jaw**

    This might look funny, but it's helpful! Right after you wake up in the morning and dash into the washroom, try out this exercise! Open your mouth, move your jaw to either side and hold for some seconds. Practice it as many times as you can.

5. **Toy with your cheeks**

    Pull either side of your cheeks out with the help of your fingers. Now use the muscles of your mouth to pull your cheeks in with your fingers still clamped to the cheeks[56]. Make sure you wash your hands before doing this exercise.

6. **Make the sound 'aaahhh'**

    Look in the mirror, open your mouth and contract the muscles of the back of your throat 30 times while you make the sound of "aaahh". Make sure you see your uvula (the dangling part in your throat) moving up and down[57]. Practice this exercise daily and become better at it because it is one of the key exercises in reducing snoring.

Once you are better at this exercise, you'll be able to move the uvula up and down without making a sound.

7. **Sing a song**

It's time to bring your inner Ed Sheeran out. This exercise is a fun one. Some of the snorers might have dreamt of becoming a singer once in life. So, you can try out singing, not professionally, but for the sake of fun and getting rid of your snoring. Singing is also a great way to have control over your throat muscles[58]. So, spend time crooning your favorite songs and stop snoring!

These exercises and remedies have been reported as the most effective. Remember, you won't see the effects and results instantly, but practicing these daily can surely make a difference in your problem. To score better chances at success, repeat the hacks consistently and set aside a few minutes of your day for exercising.

End snoring through drugstore cure & gadgets

-Neil deGrasse Tyson

Snoring is so common in the world that you'll not be amazed if we tell you that there are anti-snoring kits available in the market. Yes, a complete kit that has some pieces to stop your snoring. Generally, these kits include some chewing tablets or gums, a throat, and a nasal spray. It's natural and active ingredients focus on shrinking down the soft, swollen tissues in your throat that blocks your nasal passage[59].

By now, you've probably realized that your snoring may be a cause for concern not only for you but also the ones around you. So, it's final that it has to stop one way or the other.

Every now and then we tend to jump to medicines for the cure of any disease. This is simply because medicines are the easiest, simplest, and quickest option to eliminate any disease. People who are under this disease exhibit no different behavior to the use of drugs. Most of you people might be reading this book to find out the best over the counter products for their disease. Let's make it interesting for those who are here to find out what works best.

First up, we have some over-the-counter (OCT) products. Nasal abnormalities can be real, and a lot of snoring is due to congestions. A variety of products are designed to treat the nasal congestions that are a probable cause of snoring[60]. Some nasal support devices may relieve you from intense snoring. The most popular device is **nasal dilator**, which is a tiny snore pin, and according to satisfied customers, it really has a significant impact on snoring. Two comes in each package and are for $15. To shut down your snoring, another one available in the market is a **chinstrap**; this will force you to breathe through your nose and keep your mouth shut. Comparatively it is less expensive and handy; only for $10, you can put a stop to your snoring[61].

There are some snoring strips too, that helps you breathe easily and can drop your snoring significantly down. These breathing strips keep the flow of air smooth, and the nasal passages open[62]. They move apart your nostrils a little apart, creating more passage for air to pass out[63]. **Breathe right nasal strips** are just like a bandage, stick it on the bridge of your nose, and it will keep your nasal passage open. Great for congested nose, you cannot judge their cost and effectiveness. The price of these nasal strips ranges from $5-$40.

The next device that is a popular anti-snoring product is lubricating spray. Yes, like your machines and doors need lubrication to work properly, same goes for snoring. Lubricating sprays usually moisturize the throat to minimize snoring. However, more than dry throats blocked airways are the real cause of snoring, but the minty flavor in the lubricating spray may help clear up your chest or nasal congestion, which can minimize snoring. Some of the best anti-snoring sprays include Nytol anti-snoring throat spray, Profesnore, Asonor, Snorezee[64]. These snoring sprays can cost you anything between $15 to $50[65].

Other products include some pills and herbal medicines that claim to reduce it, but these haven't been adequately studied[66].

Some oral appliances or gadgets are mouth guard and retainers that can be inserted in the mouth while you are asleep. They prevent the collapse of the airways responsible for making this awful sound of snoring that we hear at night[67]. Some best and easily available oral retainers on the market are SnoreRX, ZQuiet, and Vitalsleep. These retainers or oral devices are a little costly, and they may cost you anything between $50-$170[68].

If there is one type of product that is very popular and does well with this problem, it is snoring pillows. Here's how an anti-snoring pillow is different from a normal pillow:

Normal pillow

- While a normal pillow will just provide you comfort and support to your neck, an anti-snoring pillow will make sure that you don't disturb your partner's sleep.

- Normal pillows are best to cuddle with, but they are definitely not going to help you in putting a stop to your snoring.

- Super comfortable and mushy, a normal pillow does not have any sensors placed in it to discern when a person is snoring.

- Anti-snoring pillows are specifically designed to stifle the harsh snoring sounds for as long as you sleep.

- pillows are extremely comfortable while you lie on your side on these pillows. These are just to aid you to sleep on your side without making you uncomfortable at all.

- Most of these pillows have a hose attached to them with sensors that sense when the person is snoring; they immediately inflate gently to adjust your head to a sleeping position that does not make you snore[69].

The problem with these OTC products is that they are uncomfortable to use, specially the oral devices so they can keep you awake all night, making you sleep deprived which is malicious for your health[70]. Also, there are enough over-the-counter products available in the market to make you confuse which one to try out. The process may involve some experimenting before you finally get rid of snoring. However, they have no side effects or bear no aftermaths so you can try for once.

If you have read carefully and paid heed to whatever was written, you might have noticed that somehow the problem lies with the nasal passages, and most of these gadgets, devices, and cures are directed towards it. Therefore, if you keep your nasal and throat passage clear, chances are higher, you can finally say bye to snoring.

These devices and products are easily available at online portals such as amazon.com, tuck.com, vital sleep.com[71]. They have completely written descriptions of these devices. Some of you might find these devices pricy, but this is the least expensive option after home remedies, that doesn't work for everyone. Other than the online portals, you can find them in nearby stores too.

If these workouts and these gadgets doesn't help you, you need professional advice from a doctor. Often it seems so difficult to make this decision, but you already made two steps: You know something is not alright and you tried to solve on your own. Now is the right time to take the next step and get advice from a doctor. What advices could he give you? Maybe you need to train more, but if you tried it for some time, it looks like he will explain you what the alternatives are.

Caution: Before trying out any of these products, make sure you consult your doctor and ask him to prescribe you the best cure.

Surgeries to cure snoring

While many of you might be very much pleased with the results of home remedies and devices mentioned above, some of you might wonder what benefit they had because they did nothing for them. These over-the-counter products, though easily available in the market, does not guarantee oh so amazing results. The reason behind this paradox is that they suffer through chronic snoring, and those devices are not actually meant for them. They have a long-term relation with this nuisance that needs to be treated with a hard-core cure.

For harsh snoring or snoring caused due to sleep apnea, doctors recommend surgical procedures when all other effective methods fail to deliver the results[72]. We shall dive into the details of these surgical procedures to know how effective they are because going for surgery might be the last choice you are left with.

Pay attention to these names; you might hear them from your doctor.

Palatal surgery/ implant

The surgery is also called the pillar procedure and is an implant. This type of minor surgery used to treat snoring and does not severe cases of sleep apnea. During this surgery, small polyester (plastic) rods are implanted into the soft upper palate of your mouth. Each of these mini implants is about 18 mm long and 1.5 mm in diameter. The palate solidifies as the tissue around these grafts heals. This way, the tissue stays more rigid and is less likely to vibrate making you snore[73].

Palatal surgery usually costs between A $2,000-3,000, and this cost includes surgery, anesthesia, and hospital or surgery day charges. This form of treatment is only effective when an oversized and droopy uvula is the cause of the snoring[74].

The overall effectiveness or success rate of this surgery remains limited, as the chances are higher if and only if appropriate patients undergo this surgery[75].

A physical deformity, which in the case of snoring, is in your nose, cause blockage of breathing, which we know is also termed as, Obstructive Sleep Apnea. If it's severe, the doctor may recommend Septoplasty or turbinate reduction surgery.

As the name implies, a turbinate reduction decreases the size of tissues inside your nose. This helps moisten as well as warm the air you breathe. Septoplasty, whilst, involves straightening of the bones and tissues placed naturally in the center of your nose. These surgeries are done together, usually one after the other[76].

Turbinate reduction/ Septoplasty is not as costly as compare to palatal implants. They may cost a patient around $800 and $10,000. It's cost largely depends on how much tissue is removed from the throat and how long the removal process takes. With insurance, the cost may increase a little say a few hundred dollars, or even free, depending on your insurance company and health plan[77].

The long-term evaluation of the surgery divulged that 68% patients experienced "improved nasal breathing" out of a total 40 patients who underwent this surgery, and eleven years after the surgery, 56% were satisfied with the overall outcome in their snoring behavior[78].

Uvulopalatopharyngoplasty (UPPP)

Yes, the name of this surgery might want you to twist your mouth a bit. But it works! This surgical procedure is done under local anesthesia, and it involves getting rid of some soft tissues attached on the back and top of the throat. In the list or removing also comes the uvula, the dangling piece of meat hanging in your throat, as well as some of the walls and palate.

This is a rare surgery, and its list of long-term side effects is intimidating. Chewing and swallowing problem tops the list of side effects. Change in voice or the permanent feeling of something in your throat are very common issues after you had gone through this surgery. For example, in a record of 186 persons the probable number of patients who can experience a change in their voice is, 15 which makes 12%, who can have swallowing problems is 26, which is 20%, and those who can undergo oral cavity is 15 which again makes 12%[79].

Some surgeons also use radiofrequency (RF) energy to remove tissues. When a laser is used during this surgery, it's called laser-assisted uvulopalatoplasty. This procedure is exclusively for treating snoring, unlike others that helped with obstructive sleep apnea too[80].

Since we know that the cost of surgeries varies greatly, same goes for this one too. Uvulopalatopharyngoplasty will cost you around $2,000 – $3,000 assisted with laser. If the surgical procedure only involved removing the uvula, it can cost you as low as $2,000. In case your snoring stems from issues with your tonsils or adenoids, the cost can be $10,000 or more without insurance[81].

According to a prospective study, the effective results 12 months post-surgery were found to be 55.6%[82].

Hypoglossal nerve stimulation

By now, it has been mentioned many times in the book that the real cause of snoring is the obstruction in the airways. And all these devices are somehow addressing the same. Hypoglossal nerve is a device directed to stimulate the nerve that has control over the upper airway passage. It has sensors that activate during sleep and sense when the person wearing it is not breathing normally[83]. Simple solution for your not so simple snoring issue!

The placement of this device in the hypoglossal nerve is by far the most expensive surgery. This surgery can cost the patient about $30,000 to $40,000, with the inclusion of hospital expenses and those associated with surgery. In the case of battery replacement of the device, the patient may need to spend extra $17,000[84].

6 months post-surgery, the results were not found to be as effective because of the technical effects that led to the dysfunction of the device[85].

Genioglossus advancement

This surgery is comparatively extensive and involves pulling forward the tongue muscle that is attached to the lower jaw. This way the tongue stays firmer and relaxes less during sleep.

This involves cutting a small piece of bone in the lower jaw where the tongue attaches, and then pull it forward. The doctor attaches the piece of bone to the lower jaw with a small screw or plate to hold the bone in place[86].

The cost of Genioglossus advancement surgery is $2,000-$10,000. Normally, insurance covers a portion of this procedure, but if not, then you may have to bear this cost all alone[87]. Looking at the success chances of this surgery, they are soaring in comparison to other surgeries. The success rate 12 months post-surgery is 95.8% of UPPP+GA[88].

Hyoid suspension

A hyoid suspension surgery requires the surgeon to move forward the elastic throat tissue, commonly known as epiglottis and the base of the tongue. This deeply opens the breathing passage.

With a deep cut into the upper throat, a surgeon detaches several tendons and some muscle. Once the hyoid bone is moved forward, a surgeon attaches it back into its place. The surgery does not affect the vocal cords; therefore, free yourself from the apprehension of having your voice changed after surgery[89].

More complex and often less effective, according to a study conducted on a group as small as 29 participants, the success rate of this surgery is found to be only 17%[90].

The surgery is also known as "hyoid myotomy and suspension" or "hyoid advancement" and is inexpensive and cost almost a fraction of the cost of complex hypoglossal nerve stimulation (HGN) implants[91].

All the above-mentioned surgeries and their cost will depend on your surgeon, the hospital you have your procedure, the length of your stay in the hospital, and what type of anesthesia will be administered during your operation[92]. It is also important to note that all these surgical procedures require extreme care and consistent post-operative checkups for at least a month.

Already thinking which surgery is best among all of the above? Well, there isn't a definite answer to this question because it largely depends on your snoring and sleeping symptoms, and only a professional doctor can tell you so.

It's clear that there are way too many surgical options to treat snoring, but that doesn't mean that they are certainly an acceptable choice for you. It is always better to consider all the choices and remedies beforehand because no surgery guarantees solving your stubborn snoring permanently and all of these come with inherent risks. Moreover, prodding your organs with a knife for no reason is always a risk. Alarming, isn't it? Try to get a second opinion from another doctor. And don't be shy to ask as many questions as possible, because it is your life and you want to get all the information you need to make such a hard decision like surgery. Additionally, think of it as your last option before just getting under the knife.

Conclusion

Snoring is a problem that is common to a wide range of people, and almost everyone knows or has heard of someone who snores. 1 in 3 of all men snore, and 1 in 4 of all women snore. This is a high number, and as such, it is a pertinent problem that needs to be addressed. People who snore have found that not only do they suffer through the embarrassment of the ridicule and mockery that others put them through, but they also find themselves at risk of losing important relationships with people that they tend to share a bed with.

A snorer experiences a lot in his or her life just because of a problem that he or she didn't even realize they had until someone else pointed it to them. Snoring comes about due to the vibration of the respiratory structure caused by the obstruction in the passage of air through the nose or throat or both. This is a vibration that produces sound like any other, but this particular one, despite it being a somewhat normal occurrence causes embarrassment to the person who let out the sound. You, as a snorer are then seen as a nuisance and a disturbance to people who are affected by it. This is really no ideal way to live.

Snoring is most often confused with Sleep apnea. Distinguishing between these two is the key to curing this condition and getting rid of the nightmare that is snoring. Snoring is basically just a vibration, creating a sound, meanwhile sleep apnea is a condition with loud and frequent snores as its signs. Sleep apnea, on its own is made of two types. Obstructive sleep apnea is the blockage or pause in breathing due to the collapse or narrowing of the upper airway. Most often here, the person has to wake up from sleep often to catch his breath, and this comes out as loud snores. Waking up doesn't happen in normal snoring. This waking up during the night disrupts sleep, and this makes you not to be able to sleep well, and people suffering from this type of sleep apnea are almost always found to be very tired during the day as they didn't get enough sleep during the night.

The other type of sleep apnea is central sleep apnea, and this is not very common. This type doesn't block the airway, but vibrations are caused due to the brain not being able to send signals to the muscles to breathe. Mostly the lower brain is affected. From Obstructive sleep apnea, it is easy to understand why it can be confused with snoring.

Not to worry, you can easily know if you have these conditions so that you can be treated. While you can monitor if you snore through your partner or someone you share a bed or room with, or some phone apps, some significant signs of sleep apnea could be fatigue and tiredness, mood swings and forgetfulness, gaping sensations and choking, waking up with a dry or sore throat, loud snoring, recurrent awakenings and headaches.

Snoring is a very common phenomenon, but that doesn't erase its negative consequences. So many people snore, and there are many factors that influence this. While increase in age increases the incidence of snoring as explained in the paragraphs above, this doesn't mean that young people don't suffer from snoring as well. When you take outage, other factors that cause snoring could be gaining excess weight, use of some extra medication, a rapidly declining immunity, dehydration, sleep deprivation, obesity, alcohol, booze, and tobacco, etc. While these could cause snoring, there are always other factors that are medically related that cause snoring. These are; gender, as we see above, pregnancy, heart disease or high cholesterol levels, allergy, congestion and nasal structure, abnormality in carotid artery, and genetic factors.

These are a lot, but the good news is there are solutions for snoring. These are; some apps on the internet like Sore lab, Snore report etc., anti-snore pillows, cleaning airway with saline before bed, exercises on your airway muscles like tongue curlers, pronouncing words, shutting your mouth for a bit, moving your jaw, toying with your cheeks etc., some drugs and some gadgets, and even in extreme cases, different kinds of surgery.

If you are reading this book, you have already taken the responsibility for your problem, and that is a good thing. Snoring is like a sprained ankle that you can make better by improving and treating. You need to train for a bit to be able to have results and your result is better sleep for you and those around you. You are never alone; all you need is for you to talk about your problem. Don't be embarrassed. You can take care of it. Always speak to a doctor or specialist about a problem, and even before using any of the solutions, make sure you consult your doctor or specialist first. Do all this, and in no time, you will be in top form. Congratulations on your first step at trying to get rid of your problem.

Sources

[1]   Jeanne Segal, Ph.D., Melinda Smith, M.A., Lawrence Robinson, and Robert Segal, M.A. (2019): How to Stop Snoring. Edited by Helpguideorg International. Available online at www.helpguide.org/articles/sleep/snoring-tips-to-help-you-and-your-partner-sleep-better.htm/, updated on June 2019, checked on 7/10/2019.

[2]   https://www.sleepfoundation.org/sites/default/files/inline-files/2005_summary_of_findings.pdf#page=31

[3]   NATIONAL SLEEP FOUNDATION (2019): Lack of Sleep is Affecting Americans, Finds the National Sleep Foundation. NATIONAL SLEEP FOUNDATION. Available online at https://www.sleepfoundation.org/press-release/lack-sleep-affecting-americans-finds-national-sleep-foundation, checked on 10/11/2019.

[4]   Cleveland Clinic (2014): Snoring. Possible Causes. Edited by Cleveland Clinic. Available online at https://my.clevelandclinic.org/health/symptoms/15580-snoring/possible-causes, updated on 8/25/2014, checked on 9/10/2019.

[5]   Siamak N. Nabili, MD, MPH; Jay W. Marks, M. D. (2018): Snoring Causes, Aids, Remedies, Solutions. Snoring definition and facts. Edited by MedicineNet. Available online at https://www.medicinenet.com/snoring/article.htm#snoring_definition_and_facts, updated on 11/8/2018, checked on 9/1/2019.

[6]   Siamak N. Nabili, MD, MPH; Jay W. Marks, M. D. (2018): Snoring Causes, Aids, Remedies, Solutions. What cause snoring. Edited by MedicineNet. Available online at https://www.medicinenet.com/snoring/article.htm#snoring_definition_and_facts, updated on 11/8/2018, checked on 9/1/2019.

[7]   Markham Heid (2019): Is Snoring Dangerous? Here's When to Worry. Edited by TIME USA. Available online at https://time.com/5491944/what-causes-snoring/, checked on 7/12/2019.

[8]   Young T, Evans L, Finn L, Palta M. Estimation of the clinically diagnosed proportion of sleep apnea syndrome in middle-aged men and women. Sleep 1997;20(9):705-6.

[9]   American Sleep Apnea Association (n.d.): Is it snoring or sleep apnea. American Sleep Apnea Association. Available online at https://www.sleepapnea.org/learn/sleep-apnea/do-i-have-sleep-apnea/is-it-snoring-or-sleep-apnea/, checked on 10/3/2019.

[10]   Kevin Asp (2017): Obstructive vs. Central Sleep Apnea. Key Differences and Treatment Options. AAST. Available online at https://www.aastweb.org/blog/obstructive-vs.-central-sleep-apnea-key-differences-and-treatment-options, checked on 9/15/2019.

[11]   Mayo Clinic (2019): Obstructive sleep apnea. Mayo Clinic. Available online at https://www.mayoclinic.org/diseases-conditions/obstructive-sleep-apnea/symptoms-causes/syc-20352090, checked on 9/15/2019.

[12]   American Sleep Apnea Association (n.d.): Is it snoring or sleep apnea. American Sleep Apnea Association. Available online at https://www.sleepapnea.org/learn/sleep-apnea/do-i-have-sleep-apnea/is-it-snoring-or-sleep-apnea/, checked on 10/3/2019.

[13]   SDA Editorial Staff (2018): How Do You Know You Snore If You Live Alone? Edited by The Sleep Guardian. Available online at https://sleepguardian.com.au/blogs/news/how-do-you-know-you-snore-if-you-live-alone, checked on 10/15/2019.

[14]   Rachael Rettner (2017): Sleep Apnea: Symptoms, Causes and Treatments. Future US, Inc. Available online at https://www.livescience.com/34797-sleep-apnea.html, checked on 7/10/2019.

[15]   NDTV Convergence Limited (2019): Do You Have Sleep Apnoea? Know The Symptoms; It May Cause Memory Loss, Depression. NDTV Convergence Limited. Available online at https://www.ndtv.com/health/do-you-have-sleep-apnoea-know-the-symptoms-it-may-cause-memory-loss-depression-1989919, updated on 2/7/2019, checked on 10/10/2019.

[16]   Mayo Clinic (2019): Obstructive sleep apnea. Mayo Clinic. Available online at https://www.mayoclinic.org/diseases-conditions/obstructive-sleep-apnea/symptoms-causes/syc-20352090, checked on 9/15/2019.

17   Melinda Ratini, DO, MS (2018): Obstructive Sleep Apnea Explained. WebMD LLC. Available online at https://www.webmd.com/sleep-disorders/guide/understanding-obstructive-sleep-apnea-syndrome#1, checked on 9/21/2019.

18   Arthur Allen (2014): Clues You Might Have Obstructive Sleep Apnea. WebMD LLC. Available online at https://www.webmd.com/sleep-disorders/sleep-apnea/features/sleep-apnea-clues#1, checked on 6/5/2019.

19   American Migraine Foundation (2019): Sleep Disorders and Headache. American Migraine Foundation. Available online at https://americanmigrainefoundation.org/resource-library/sleep/, updated on 4/8/2019, checked on 10/10/2019.

20   Markham Heid (2019): Is Snoring Dangerous? Here's When to Worry. Edited by TIME USA. Available online at https://time.com/5491944/what-causes-snoring/, checked on 7/12/2019.

21   NATIONAL SLEEP FOUNDATION (2019): Lack of Sleep is Affecting Americans, Finds the National Sleep Foundation. NATIONAL SLEEP FOUNDATION. Available online at https://www.sleepfoundation.org/press-release/lack-sleep-affecting-americans-finds-national-sleep-foundation, checked on 10/11/2019.

22   Yagana Shah (2015): Why You Snore More As You Get Older And What You Can Do About It. Verizon Media. Available online at https://www.huffpost.com/entry/how-to-stop-snoring_n_7687906?guccounter=1, updated on 12/6/2017, checked on 6/25/2019.

23   Louise Chang, M. D. (2018): The Basics of Snoring. WebMD LLC. Available online at https://www.webmd.com/sleep-disorders/guide/snoring, checked on 7/5/2019.

24   Sarah Stevenson (2019): A Loss of Appetite in the Elderly. A Place for Mom, Inc. Available online at https://www.aplaceformom.com/blog/01-23-2013-loss-of-appetite-in-elderly/, checked on 9/20/2019.

25   Leslie Kernisan (2015): A Geriatrician's Advice on Sleep Problems and Dementia. A Place for Mom, Inc. Available online at https://www.aplaceformom.com/blog/11-26-15-manage-sleep-problems-in-dementia/, checked on 6/25/2019.

26   Moein Foroughi, Hossein Razavi, Majid Malekmohammad, Parisa Adimi Naghan, Hamidreza Jamaati (2016): Diagnosis of Obstructive Sleep Apnea Syndrome in Adults: A Brief Review of Existing Data for Practice in Iran. National Research Institute of Tuberculosis and Lung Disease. Available online at https://www.ncbi.nlm.nih.gov/pmc/articles/PMC5127617/, checked on 9/7/2019.

27   Jeanne Segal, Ph.D., Melinda Smith, M.A., Lawrence Robinson, and Robert Segal, M.A. (2019): How to Stop Snoring. Edited by Helpguideorg International. Available online at www.helpguide.org/articles/sleep/snoring-tips-to-help-you-and-your-partner-sleep-better.htm/, updated on June 2019, checked on 7/10/2019.

28   Yvette Brazier, Natalie Olsen (2018): Measuring BMI for adults, children, and teens. Healthline Media UK Ltd. Available online at https://www.medicalnewstoday.com/articles/323622.php, checked on 6/18/2019.

29   Centers for Disease Control and Prevention (2015): Assessing Your Weight. Centers for Disease Control and Prevention. Available online at https://www.cdc.gov/healthyweight/assessing/index.html, checked on 6/10/2019.

30   https://www.ncbi.nlm.nih.gov/pmc/articles/PMC3644827/

31   Jeanne Segal, Ph.D., Melinda Smith, M.A., Lawrence Robinson, and Robert Segal, M.A. (2019): How to Stop Snoring. Edited by Helpguideorg International. Available online at www.helpguide.org/articles/sleep/snoring-tips-to-help-you-and-your-partner-sleep-better.htm/, updated on June 2019, checked on 7/10/2019.

32   Austin Frakt (2017): How Many Pills Are Too Many? New York Times Company. Available online at https://www.nytimes.com/2017/04/10/upshot/how-many-pills-are-too-many.html, checked on 9/10/2019.

33   Siamak N. Nabili, MD, MPH; Jay W. Marks, M. D. (2018): Snoring Causes, Aids, Remedies, Solutions. Snoring definition and facts. Edited by MedicineNet. Available online at https://www.medicinenet.com/snoring/article.htm#snoring_definition_and_facts, updated on

34   Harvard University (2015): Snoring solutions. Simple changes can help to turn down the volume. Harvard University, updated on https://www.health.harvard.edu/diseases-and-conditions/snoring-solutions, checked on 6/15/2019.

35   SnoreLab (n.d.): Age and Snoring. Edited by SnoreLab. Available online at https://www.snorelab.com/age-and-snoring/, checked on 10/17/2019.

[36] Amy Marturana (2017): 7 Common Causes of Dry Mouth—and How to Fix It. Condé Nast. Available online at https://www.self.com/story/causes-of-dry-mouth-and-dry-mouth-remedies, checked on 9/1/2019.

[37] TUCK.COM LLC (2019): How Much Sleep Does a Person Need? TUCK.COM LLC. Available online at https://www.tuck.com/how-much-sleep-do-i-need/, checked on 6/14/2019.

[38] Siamak N. Nabili, MD, MPH; Jay W. Marks, M. D. (2018): Snoring Causes, Aids, Remedies, Solutions. Snoring definition and facts. Edited by MedicineNet. Available online at https://www.medicinenet.com/snoring/article.htm#snoring_definition_and_facts, updated on Medical conditions / causes triggering snoring

[39] Emily Gurnon (2018): Why Snoring Gets Worse With Age and What You Can Do About It. Next Avenue. Available online at https://www.nextavenue.org/why-snoring-gets-worse-with-age-and-what-you-can-do-about-it/, checked on 8/15/2019.

[40] Ashley Marcin; Mark R Laflamme (2016): Is There a Link Between Cholesterol and Sleep? Healthline Media. Available online at https://www.healthline.com/health/high-cholesterol/sleep-and-cholesterol#1, checked on 9/4/2019.

[41] https://www.ncbi.nlm.nih.gov/pmc/articles/PMC3627372/

[42] Northwestern University (n.d.): What Are Nasal Deformities? Northwestern University. Available online at https://www.nm.org/conditions-and-care-areas/ent-ear-nose-throat/nasal-deformity, checked on 8/22/2019.

[43] Christian Nordqvist (2013): Snoring Can Affect The Carotid Artery. Edited by Healthline Media UK Ltd. Available online at https://www.medicalnewstoday.com/articles/255459.php, checked on 9/1/2019.

[44] Victor Hoffstein (n.d.): Snoring and Sleep. NATIONAL SLEEP FOUNDATION. Available online at https://www.sleepfoundation.org/articles/snoring-and-sleep, checked on 8/15/2019.

[45] Kyra Oliver (2017): How to Stop Snoring – 11 Remedies that Work! Dr. Axe. Available online at https://draxe.com/health/how-to-stop-snoring/, checked on 6/14/2019.

[46] Dr Mike Dilkes (2017): How to stop snoring in just five minutes a day. Top ear, nose and throat consultant reveals the secret to a peaceful night's sleep in new book. Associated Newspapers Ltd. Available online at https://www.dailymail.co.uk/health/article-4889158/Snoring-stopped-five-minutes-day-exercises.html, checked on 8/23/2019.

[47] Jeanne Segal, Ph.D., Melinda Smith, M.A., Lawrence Robinson, and Robert Segal, M.A. (2019): How to Stop Snoring. Edited by Helpguideorg International. Available online at www.helpguide.org/articles/sleep/snoring-tips-to-help-you-and-your-partner-sleep-better.htm/, updated on June 2019, checked on 7/10/2019.

[48] Linda Melone; Louise Chang, M. D. (2012): 7 Easy Fixes for Snoring. Edited by WebMD LLC. Available online at https://www.webmd.com/sleep-disorders/features/easy-snoring-remedies#1, checked on 9/23/2019.

[49] Erica Cirino; Elaine K. Luo, M. D. (2017): 15 Remedies That Will Stop Snoring. Edited by Healthline Media. Available online at https://www.healthline.com/health/snoring-remedies#remedies, checked on 8/10/2019.

[50] Maria Cassano (2016): How To Stop Snoring At Night, According To A Snoring Expert. Bustle Company. Available online at https://www.bustle.com/articles/173851-how-to-stop-snoring-at-night-according-to-a-snoring-expert, checked on 8/10/2019.

[51] Louise Chang, M. D. (2012): 7 Easy Fixes for Snoring. WebMD LLC. Available online at https://www.webmd.com/sleep-disorders/features/easy-snoring-remedies#2, checked on 10/10/2019.

[52] Daniel Ayer (2019): 8 Foods that Cause Snoring: Avoid These at All Costs! Snoring Source. Available online at https://www.snoringsource.com/can-food-cause-snoring/, checked on 10/10/2019.

[53] SnoreLab (n.d.): Mouth Exercises for Snoring. Edited by SnoreLab. Available online at https://www.snorelab.com/mouth-exercises-for-snoring/, checked on 9/10/2019.

[54] Jan Wrede (2017): Exercises to Stop Snoring. What Really Works? Edited by somnishop.net. Available online at https://somnishop.net/exercises-to-stop-snoring-what-really-works/, checked on 7/10/2019.

55   Jeanne Segal, Ph.D., Melinda Smith, M.A., Lawrence Robinson, and Robert Segal, M.A. (2019): How to Stop Snoring. Edited by Helpguideorg International. Available online at www.helpguide.org/articles/sleep/snoring-tips-to-help-you-and-your-partner-sleep-better.htm/, updated on June 2019, checked on 7/10/2019.

56   Jan Wrede (2017): Exercises to Stop Snoring. What Really Works? Edited by somnishop.net. Available online at https://somnishop.net/exercises-to-stop-snoring-what-really-works/, checked on 7/10/2019.

57   Jeanne Segal, Ph.D., Melinda Smith, M.A., Lawrence Robinson, and Robert Segal, M.A. (2019): How to Stop Snoring. Edited by Helpguideorg International. Available online at www.helpguide.org/articles/sleep/snoring-tips-to-help-you-and-your-partner-sleep-better.htm/, updated on June 2019, checked on 7/10/2019.

58   Elizabeth Brown (2017): I Tried Five Products to Stop Snoring and Some Kind of Worked. There was drool, fear, and in one case, quieter sleep. Vice media group. Available online at https://www.vice.com/en_us/article/59y4vq/products-to-stop-snoring, checked on 9/27/2019.

59   William Blahd, M. D. (2017): Understanding Snoring -- Diagnosis and Treatment. Edited by WebMD LLC. Available online at https://www.webmd.com/sleep-disorders/understanding-snoring-treatment#1, checked on 10/17/2019.

60   Julie Evans, Richard N. Fogoros, MD (2019): The 7 Best Anti-Snoring Devices of 2019. Dotdash publishing, updated on https://www.verywellhealth.com/best-anti-snoring-devices-4686087, checked on 22 October.

61   Lisa Esposito (2015): What Works for Snoring? U.S. News & World Report L.P. Available online at https://health.usnews.com/health-news/health-wellness/articles/2015/06/16/what-works-for-snoring, checked on 8 Aufust 2019.

62   Jae Curtis (n.d.): Snoring Aids: Do They Really Work? Edited by Colgate-Palmolive Company. Available online at https://www.colgate.com/en-us/oral-health/conditions/respiratory-conditions/snoring-aids-do-they-really-work-0214, checked on 9/5/2019.

63   Julie Evans, Richard N. Fogoros, MD (2019): The 7 Best Anti-Snoring Devices of 2019. Dotdash publishing, updated on https://www.verywellhealth.com/best-anti-snoring-devices-4686087, checked on 22 October.

64   Jae Curtis (n.d.): Snoring Aids: Do They Really Work? Edited by Colgate-Palmolive Company. Available online at https://www.colgate.com/en-us/oral-health/conditions/respiratory-conditions/snoring-aids-do-they-really-work-0214, checked on 9/5/2019.

65   amazon.co.uk/d/Nasal-Strips-Breathing-Aids/Nytol-Anti-Snoring-Throat-Spray-50ml/B00C7P6YWO

66   exsnorer.org (n.d.): A List of The Best Anti-Snoring Sprays from 2018 for Snoring Relief. exsnorer.org. Available online at https://www.exsnorer.org/anti-snoring-sprays-ultimate-guide/, checked on 9/25/2019.

67   William Blahd, M. D. (2017): Understanding Snoring -- Diagnosis and Treatment. Edited by WebMD LLC. Available online at https://www.webmd.com/sleep-disorders/understanding-snoring-treatment#1, checked on 10/17/2019.

68   Jae Curtis (n.d.): Snoring Aids: Do They Really Work? Edited by Colgate-Palmolive Company. Available online at https://www.colgate.com/en-us/oral-health/conditions/respiratory-conditions/snoring-aids-do-they-really-work-0214, checked on 9/5/2019.

69   Dennis James (n.d.): 10 Best Anti-Snoring Devices That Will Actually Quiet You Down. Snore Mentor. Available online at https://www.snorementor.com/best-anti-snoring-devices-aids/, checked on 9/25/2019.

70   Elizabeth Brown (2017): I Tried Five Products to Stop Snoring and Some Kind of Worked. There was drool, fear, and in one case, quieter sleep. Vice media group. Available online at https://www.vice.com/en_us/article/59y4vq/products-to-stop-snoring, checked on 9/27/2019.

71   William Blahd, M. D. (2017): Understanding Snoring -- Diagnosis and Treatment. Edited by WebMD LLC. Available online at https://www.webmd.com/sleep-disorders/understanding-snoring-treatment#1, checked on 10/17/2019.

72   Jae Curtis (n.d.): Snoring Aids: Do They Really Work? Edited by Colgate-Palmolive Company. Available online at https://www.colgate.com/en-us/oral-health/conditions/respiratory-conditions/snoring-aids-do-they-really-work-0214, checked on 9/5/2019.

[73]   Erica Cirino (2018): Surgical Options to Treat the Causes of Excessive Snoring. Edited by Healthline Media. Available online at https://www.healthline.com/health/surgery-for-snoring#summary, checked on 10/1/2019.

[74]   The Sleep Therapy Clinic Pty Ltd (n.d.): Surgical Treatments For Snoring And Apnoea. The Sleep Therapy Clinic Pty Ltd. Available online at http://www.sleeptherapyclinic.com.au/surgical-treatments-snoring-apnoea-apnea, checked on 7/18/2019.

[75]   Oğuz Kuşcu, Rıza Önder Günaydın, Tevfik Sözen, Münir Demir Bajin, Oğuz Öğretmenoğlu (2014): Which Patients Can Benefit from Pillar Palatal Implant Procedure? Turk Arch Otolaryngol (52: 93-7). Available online at: https://pdfs.semanticscholar.org/6071/500a7fb3d7c98abf9c9131d8f79670317067.pdf, checked on 7/10/2019.

[76]   Erica Cirino (2018): Surgical Options to Treat the Causes of Excessive Snoring. Edited by Healthline Media. Available online at https://www.healthline.com/health/surgery-for-snoring#summary, checked on 10/1/2019.

[77]   Erica Cirino, Daniel Murrell, MD (2018): Turbinate Reduction: What to Expect. Healthline Media. Available online at https://www.healthline.com/health/turbinate-reduction#cost, checked on 9/15/2019.

[78]   https://www.ncbi.nlm.nih.gov/pmc/articles/PMC6033599/

[79]   Maria Värendh; Sören Berg; Morgan Andersson (2012): Long-term follow-up of patients operated with Uvulopalatopharyngoplasty from 1985 to 1991. Elsevier Ltd. Available online at https://www.sciencedirect.com/science/article/pii/S0954611112003514, checked on 9/28/2019.

[80]   Erica Cirino (2018): Surgical Options to Treat the Causes of Excessive Snoring. Edited by Healthline Media. Available online at https://www.healthline.com/health/surgery-for-snoring#summary, checked on 10/1/2019.

[81]   Robert J. Hudson (n.d.): Snoring Surgery Cost and Insurance Answers. SnoreNation. Available online at https://snorenation.com/snoring-surgery-cost-insurance-answers/, checked on 10/20/2019.

[82]   https://www.ncbi.nlm.nih.gov/pmc/articles/PMC4451538/

[83]   Brandon Peters (2019): Electronic Tongue Device for Sleep Apnea. Implanted Hypoglossal Nerve Stimulator Helps Open Airway. Dotdash publishing. Available online at https://www.verywellhealth.com/hypoglossal-nerve-stimulator-for-treating-sleep-apnea-3015195, checked on 9/5/2019.

[84]   Brandon Peters (2019): Inspire Hypoglossal Nerve Stimulator Surgery for Sleep Apnea Treatment. Dotdash publishing. Available online at https://www.verywellhealth.com/inspire-for-sleep-apnea-3015288, checked on 10/26/2019.

[85]   https://www.ncbi.nlm.nih.gov/pmc/articles/PMC5610953/

[86]   Stanford Health Care (n.d.): Genioglossus Advancement. Stanford Health Care. Available online at https://stanfordhealthcare.org/medical-treatments/t/tongue-surgery/types/genioglossus-advancement.html, checked on 6/10/2019.

[87]   Dr. Schendel Plastic Surgery (n.d.): Genioglossus Advancement. Sleep Apnea Surgery. Dr. Schendel Plastic Surgery. Available online at https://schendelmd.com/procedures/sleep-disorder-surgery/genioglossus-advancement-palo-alto-ca, checked on 8/16/2019.

[88]   https://www.ncbi.nlm.nih.gov/pmc/articles/PMC4451538/

[89]   Lexington Clinic (n.d.): Hyoid Suspension. Lexington Clinic. Available online at https://www.lexingtonclinic.com/osasurgery/hyoid.html, checked on 9/17/2019.

[90]   Erica Cirino (2018): Surgical Options to Treat the Causes of Excessive Snoring. Edited by Healthline Media. Available online at https://www.healthline.com/health/surgery-for-snoring#summary, checked on 10/1/2019.

[91]   Siesta Medical, Inc (n.d.): What is Airlift? Siesta Medical, Inc. Available online at https://www.siestamedical.com/airlift-tm, checked on 9/25/2019.

[92]   Robert J. Hudson (n.d.): Snoring Surgery Cost and Insurance Answers. SnoreNation. Available online at https://snorenation.com/snoring-surgery-cost-insurance-answers/, checked on 10/20/2019.